YOUR KNOWLEDGE HAS VALUE

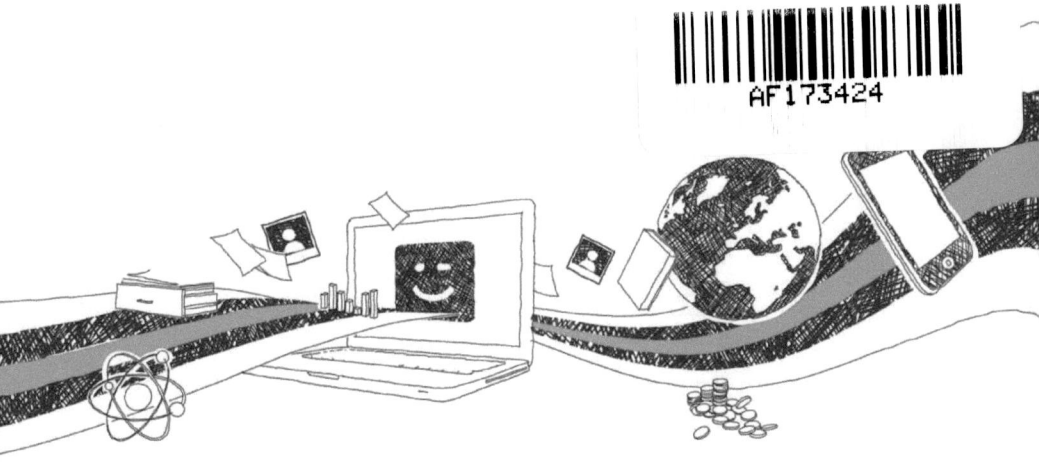

- We will publish your bachelor's and master's thesis, essays and papers

- Your own eBook and book - sold worldwide in all relevant shops

- Earn money with each sale

Upload your text at www.GRIN.com and publish for free

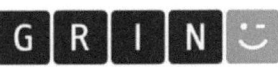

Wendy Soon

Did the brain create God, or God create the brain?

GRIN Publishing

Bibliographic information published by the German National Library:

The German National Library lists this publication in the National Bibliography;
detailed bibliographic data are available on the Internet at http://dnb.dnb.de .

Imprint:

Copyright © 2008 GRIN Verlag GmbH
Print and binding: Books on Demand GmbH, Norderstedt Germany
ISBN: 978-3-656-17610-7

This book at GRIN:

http://www.grin.com/en/e-book/192040/did-the-brain-create-god-or-god-create-
the-brain

GRIN - Your knowledge has value

Since its foundation in 1998, GRIN has specialized in publishing academic texts by students, college teachers and other academics as e-book and printed book. The website www.grin.com is an ideal platform for presenting term papers, final papers, scientific essays, dissertations and specialist books.

Visit us on the internet:

http://www.grin.com/

http://www.facebook.com/grincom

http://www.twitter.com/grin_com

Assess the claim that there is a neurophysiological basis for religious beliefs.

Introduction

Every country, every race, every people around the world have their religions, just like they have their own cultures and traditions. Although every religion evolves around different deities, different values and different practices, they all meet the same need—the need of the human race to have a meaning in life and to seek a refuge in a higher being. The fact that various groups of human beings with distinctly different lifestyles and cultures actually have this consistency of having a religion brings to attention that religion may in fact be an inherent need of human beings. Why would religion be an inherent need? Many scientists, psychologists and philosophers have proposed that this need may be related to how the human brain has been wired, and wired to need something called 'God'.

Neurotheology is a new study that has emerged from the attempt to link religion to the brain. It is the study that unites two seemingly unrelated entities--religion and the brain--in the hopes of being able to better understand both entities. By investigating the link between the brain and religion, controversies have arisen as to whether religious experiences and God could be reduced to nothing more than the result of brain functions. This theory is termed as reductionism.

In the process of studying the brain, researchers have used high-tech brain imaging techniques to observe the neurological changes in the brain in response to different stimuli. One such technique is the single photon emission computed topography (SPECT) that visualizes brain activity by using radioactive tracers and a scanner to produce a picture of the brain. Other methods include the positron emission topography (PET) scans and functional magnetic resonance imaging (fMRI). Each of these techniques has its own advantages and limitations, such as poor spatial and temporal resolutions, as well as high noise levels.[1,33-36] Nonetheless, these brain studies have produced some consistent results as to which brain areas are stimulated and which tend to have a dramatic drop in activity during peaks of spiritual experiences. However, there is still insufficient evidence to say that there is a neurophysiological basis for religious beliefs. Any information obtained thus far merely identifies which parts of the brain are involved in spiritual experiences, but do not serve to prove that these spiritual experiences as merely a result of certain mis-firings of the brain. Furthermore, all the scientific evidence collected thus far only points to the link between the human brain and spiritual experiences, which does not equate to a link to religious beliefs.[2] Henceforth, the claim that there is a neurological basis for religious beliefs has no concrete evidences to support it and thus does not stand.

Definitions

The term basis refers to a fundamental principle or groundwork from which something else is built upon. Other synonyms for "basis" include "source", "origin", "beginning" and "foundation". As such, the claim of a neurophysiological *basis* of religious beliefs is not just a declaration of a relationship between the brain and religious beliefs, but also arguing that religious beliefs *originate* from the brain.

Religious belief is a faith or creed concerning the supernatural, sacred, or divine. It may concern the existence and worship of one or more deities. In addition to that, religious belief may also relate to the values and practices based on the teachings of a spiritual leader.[3]

Religious experience (also known as spiritual experience) is an occasion when the person in question comes into contact with transcendental reality.[4] Religious experiences are very personal encounters that may be very out of the ordinary, and thus may be received with skepticism by others. To make things worse, these experiences may be similar to those arising from psychopathological states such as psychoses and altered awareness.[5,6]

Brain functions and their proposed relation to religion

One important brain region that is involved in neurotheology is the Orientation Association Area (OAA). The primary job of the OAA is to orient the individual in physical space, and to draw a sharp distinction between the individual and everything else (the rest of the universe), giving us a sense of 'self'. Thus, during the normal state of mind, the OAA is a place of furious brain activity. A drop in activity levels in the OAA can occur during meditation or injury. This drop in activity may be due to a block in the flow of sensory information from the hippocampus to the

OAA, causing it to be unable to perform its duty properly.[7,8] When the OAA activity drops sharply, not only is there a loss of sense of self, but there is also no preferred position or direction in space, thus the local self dissolves into an omnidirectional expansion. This is often described by meditators as a "feeling of oneness with the universe".[9]

Another important brain region is the Attention Association Area (AAA), also known as the pre-frontal cortex. This region is responsible for giving the individual the ability to concentrate, plan future behavior and to carry out complex tasks that require mental focus or sustained attention. During meditation, this region is highly stimulated due to the high amount of concentration needed. Damage to this region of the brain results in the loss of ability to complete long sentences, plan a schedule, lack of will and a profound indifference to events in the environment. Victims' ability to imagine the happening of certain events is also hampered upon damage to the prefrontal cortex.[8]

It should also be mentioned that the frontal lobes and temporal lobes have also been found to be intimately connected to the limbic system that controls most of our emotions. The frontal lobes are believed to be extremely important in initiating, controlling and monitoring emotions. These areas have increased activity during the peaks of spiritual experiences, giving rise to the emotional aspects during spiritual experiences. Extensive damage to the frontal lobes usually leads to uncontrolled emotions, apathy and loss of social interests.[10,11]

The Broca's area, situated in the left frontal lobe of the brain, may be responsible for the hearing of the voice of God. Normally, we can tell if it is our inner voice that is speaking. However, when sensory information is restricted during meditation or prayer, the Broca's area may be switched on and internally generated thoughts may be misattributed to an external source.[2,9]

An important pair of sub-systems is the sympathetic system and the parasympathetic system, otherwise known as the Arousal system and the Quiescent system. These two systems are generally antagonistic to each other, but may function in a complementary manner under certain conditions. When one of these systems receives continued excessive stimulation, a "spillover" phenomenon occurs where the excessive stimulation produces activation responses in the opposite system (instead of the usual inhibitory effect). Under very rare conditions, maximal simultaneous activation of both Arousal and Quiescent systems can occur. This simultaneous activation of the two systems explains why meditation and rituals can give rise to the emotions that are often experienced. During meditation, the Quiescent system is stimulated. When the meditation reaches a peak, there is a spillover effect to the Arousal system, resulting in a spiritual "high", described by expert meditators as a "rush" or a release of energy during a hyperquiescent state. On the other hand, rhythmic rituals stimulate the Arousal system, with spillover effects to the Quiescent system, resulting in a sudden feeling of bliss, peace and oneness with the rest of the world.[2, 12]

As described above, scientific evidences have been used to explain how and why various feelings and visions are experienced during mediation and prayer. Does this then mean that neurophysiology is the absolute explanation behind spiritual experiences and, more importantly, religious beliefs? Not necessarily so.

Brain activity during religious experiences does *not* negate the existence of God

The most popular argument for the neurophysiological basis of religious beliefs is that of the detection of specific brain regions that are involved in religious experiences. However, although there has been extensive experiments conducted to figure out the link between brain activity and spiritual experiences, the classification of activity in the brain during stages of enhanced spiritual experience does not equate to the brain being the source of the experience.

The most famous of all brain experiments for this purpose is that done by Andrew Newberg and Eugene D'Aquili in Philadelphia, Pennsylvania. In their research study, Tibetan monks and Franciscan nuns well-trained in meditation were recruited. As the monks and nuns meditate, Newberg and D'Aquili sit in an adjoining room, observing their brain activity. When the observed individual approaches a transcendent peak of spiritual intensity, he or she tugs a twine that informs the researchers of the moment. Newberg and D'Aquili then take note of the brain activity of the meditator during that moment, and compare that to the previous readouts of the brain during normal states. What was mainly observed was the quieting of the OAA, which results in the feeling of proximity and oneness with God. "The absorption of the self into something larger [is] not the result of emotional fabrication or wishful thinking," Newberg and D'Aquili write in their book 'Why God Won't Go Away'. "It springs, instead, from neurological events, as when the orientation area goes dark." In a reductionist sense, this observation leads to some scientists proposing that God is thus only a creation of the brain. "The human brain has been genetically wired to encourage religious beliefs", they conclude.[2]

However, this suggestion that just because a mere association is found between specific brain activity and peaks of spiritual intensity implies that brain activity is the root of spiritual experiences, is a major fallacy. It suggests that everything we think of as reality is only a rendition of reality, merely created by the brain. Everything we observe in reality--all thoughts, feelings, memories, insights, desires, revelations--is all dependent on the processing powers of the brain, a combination of sensory perceptions and firing of neurons in the complex human brain. If this reductionist argument is true, it raises some very profound questions: not just about the neurological nature of spiritual experience, but also the most basic truths of human existence.[2, 13]

For the sake of this paper (and my own dignity), I shall assume that humans are real, and that our existence is not doubted (we are not just an imagination that was produced by the firings in the human brain). Based on this assumption, then the above argument that God is a mere creation of the brain also does not stand. Just because an experience is correlated with certain neuronal activities does not mean that the experience only exists in the brain.

Imagine you were asked to eat a slice of lemon cheesecake during an experimental study. As you savor this freshly baked cheesecake, a concurrent SPECT scan of your brain captures images of the neurological activity in the various brain regions that have been stimulated by such an activity: olfactory areas detect the wonderful aroma of lemon and Philadelphia cream cheese; visual areas perceive the sight of a golden brown graham crust topped with generous amounts of lemon flavored cream cheese; taste areas identify the rich, tangy, cheesy flavor as you sink your teeth into it. The SPECT brain scan shows all the above activity in the same way as it did during the spiritual peak of the Tibetan Buddhists and Franciscan nuns. Yet, these detections of electrical activity in the brain do not negate the reality of the lemon cheesecake you had just eaten. Instead, they merely inform us of which areas of the brain are stimulated in certain circumstances, and which areas of the brain are less involved during these actions.[2]

Similarly, the brain imaging studies only inform us of how the brain reacts during spiritual experiences, but does not give information about the cause and nature of the experience. There is indeed no way thus far to be able to determine whether the neurological changes associated with spiritual experiences are a result of the brain's own firings, or the brain reacting to a real spiritual encounter. It is merely a "proof of the existence of the brain", as neurologist James Austin puts it.[2, 14]

Spiritual experiences appear more real than baseline reality

Spiritual experiences are often compared to other events already well known to be created by the brain, such as hallucinations and dreams. The sole purpose of performing such comparisons is an attempt to judge whether spiritual experiences are as "fake" as these other experiences that originated from the brain, or if spiritual experiences are real experiences. In such an analysis, one has to first agree that reality is ultimately reducible to the vivid sense of reality, or "how real" something feels like. If this is the case, what happens when spiritual experiences are described by subjects to be more real than baseline reality, where baseline reality is the reality that comprises of our daily activities and perceptions? When we take baseline reality as the point of reference, some events would appear inferior to this baseline reality, while other events would score superiorly to baseline reality.[2] Individuals often described dreams and psychotic hallucinations as inferior to baseline reality when they reflect upon the events on retrospect. However, the same cannot be said of spiritual experiences. More often than not, individuals describe spiritual experiences to be more real than baseline reality, and such experiences often have a long lasting effect on the individual's life.[18,38] If this is true, then we have to admit that spiritual experiences are more real than baseline reality, more real than many other events in our daily lives.[33]

Reproducibility of an event does not necessarily cast doubt on its origins

Hard core subscribers to the neurological basis of religious beliefs will not accept the above repudiation of the evidence so easily. Instead, further experiments have been conducted to demonstrate the possibility of replicating experiences similar to that of spiritual experiences by triggering particular brain activities, thus attempting to strengthen the argument that the root of spiritual experiences is the human brain. The reproduction of spiritual experience can be achieved in three different manners: The administration of certain drugs; the electrical stimulation of specific brain regions; the manifestation of neural diseases or damage to specific areas of the brain.

Drugs that can create profound spiritual experiences include LSD-like indoles, substituted amphetamines, and other pharmacological agents like hallucinogenic or psychedelic drugs. Some drugs have even been used to induce spiritual experiences during religious rituals, such as the use of peyote in some Native-American groups.[15, 16] This hypothesis has been tested many years ago by Harvard professor Timothy Leary and Walter Pahnke. Leary and Pahnke gave participants psilocybin, a hallucinogen derived from mushrooms that mimics the monoamine serotonin. Not only did this drug induce a short-term mystical experience in the participants, it also caused long term effects in them. The average mysticism scores for subjects (that took psilocybin) was 64% in 1962 when the experiment was conducted, and remained at 65% 25 years later. This is significantly higher than the 14% in the matched control subjects (who took placebos) in 1962, and 13% during the follow-up.[17, 18]

Another example of drug-induced spiritual experience is the use of synthetic dimethyltryptamine (DMT), a powerful psychedelic. Volunteers injected with DMT experience overwhelming visual and emotional imagery, like an instantaneous peak of spiritual intensity. Psychiatrist Rick Strassman proposes that the body makes its own psychedelic drug. During meditation, pineal activity is enhanced, which may elicit a resonating effect with other brain regions. This harmonization resynchronizes both hemispheres of the brain, and may thus result in synergetic activity that produces hallucinogenic compounds, leading to what is known as spiritual experience. The pineal gland, also called the spirit gland, is known to contain high levels of the enzymes and building blocks that are required in the making of DMT. It may secrete DMT when inhibitory processes blocking its production are removed. DMT production is particularly stimulated during birth, sexual ecstasy, childbirth, extreme physical stress, near-death, psychosis, and physical death, as well as meditation. Thus, this endogenous source of DMT is proposed to be the clue behind spiritual experiences.[9]

Besides drugs that can induce spiritual-like experiences, there are also drugs that may be able to antagonize or alter such experiences. For example, an opiate antagonist may be used to investigate its effects on meditation and prayers. However, preliminary attempts to alter spiritual experiences thus far have been unsuccessful, suggesting that there seems to be more to spiritual experiences than just brain activity alone.[33,39]

Electrical stimulation of the brain to produce spiritual experiences (NeuroMagnetics) has been most widely studied by Michael Persinger, a professor of neuroscience at Laurentian University in Sudbury, Ontario. Persinger believed that "microseizures", due to electromagnetic fluctuations produced by solar flares, seismic activity, radio wave transmissions and even from the brain itself, are the root behind religious visions, mystical visions and even alien-abduction episodes. Persinger tested his hypothesis by using solenoids in a helmet to send electrical waves to the brains of volunteers. By bombarding different brain regions with different frequencies, different results are obtained. For example, stimulation of the amygdala produces sexual arousal; focusing the waves on the hippocampus produces an opiate effect; stimulating the temporal lobe creates sensations that volunteers describe as supernatural or spiritual. Electrical stimulation can also spillover into nearby structures, like that of the OAA and AAA as described earlier. This spillover effect may kindle the visual area to cause intense visions, or a floating feeling due to somatosensory stimulation. It is suspected that mini electrical storms in the temporal lobe can be triggered by anxiety, personal crisis, lack of oxygen and fatigue -- moments that some people 'find God'. Thus, Persinger insists that "religion is a property of the brain".[19]

The third method of reproducing spiritual experiences includes temporal-lobe epilepsy as well as some psychopathological disorders such as mania and schizophrenia. Many patients suffering from such conditions of the brain claim to experience intense spiritual phenomena.[20, 21, 22] Similarly, about a quarter of patients who have localized epileptic seizures in the temporal lobes report that they have spiritual experiences during their seizure and some even exhibit a newfound sense of religiosity after the episode. Whenever we see something that is significant to us, the message goes into the temporal lobe and is then conveyed to the limbic system, which is the brain's emotional center. Patients who have had repeated temporal lobe seizures tend to have more intense experiences when they encounter something significant to them. They are more inclined to interpret everyday occurrences as having extraordinary meaning, and often have heightened responses, particularly to religious symbols such as crosses and bibles. V.S. Ramachandran, the director of Center for Brain and Cognition at the University of California, San Diego and author of the book 'Phantoms in the Brain', explains that this phenomenon can be explained by the fact that their temporal lobes have been altered in some manner to produce heightened response to religious items, thus resulting in an enhancement of emotions related to religious or spiritual experiences. Thus he proposes that the human brain has been hard-wired with a neural circuit that specializes in mediating religious experiences.[23]

Regardless of these heightened spiritual feelings having been noted in people with psychopathological disorders, it must not be neglected that there *are* people who experience heightened emotions during a spiritual peak and are normal with no psychopathological disorders nor records of temporal lobe epilepsy.[15-16, 24-25] Not every religious person is an epileptic, and not every epileptic is religious. Hence, even though psychopathological defects may be the root of some spiritual experiences in certain individuals, the majority of such experiences cannot be explained using the psychopathological condition alone.[12, 23]

With the above suggestion that spiritual experiences can be reproduced with a variety of methods like drugs, electrical stimulation and disease, I would like to pose the question: is the reproducibility of an event equivalent to proving that the event is unreal? Definitely not. Take the simple example of weight loss. It is a widely accepted fact that one can lose weight due to various means such as exercise and dieting. A girl on a diet can feel her own weight loss by putting her hands on her waists and thus sense that they have shrunk in size. Similarly, stimulation of specific regions of the brain have been able to fool volunteers into thinking that their hands were really moving inwards and thus had shrinking waists. The study, led by Dr Henrik Ehrsson of University College London, tricked blindfolded volunteers by using gadgets that created false sensations that both hands rested on the waist were moving inwards. This success in reproducing the "shrinking feeling" does not mean that the girls can in actual fact NEVER lose weight. They can really lose weight, but this experiment merely reproduced the

sensation in them.[26] Extrapolating this to our discussion of the brain and spiritual experiences—
success in reproducing the "God" feeling does not mean that God can in actual fact NEVER
exist. God can exist, and experiments have merely served to reproduce the *feeling* of God's
presence, thus the claim that religious beliefs have a neural basis is weak.

Religious Experience is related but not equivalent to Religious Belief

All throughout the paper until this point, I have been describing scientific studies directed at
spiritual experience. However, the main question of this paper is not the neurological basis of
spiritual experiences, but the neurological basis of *religious beliefs*. Is spiritual experience equal
to religious beliefs? By taking a second look at the definitions of these two terms earlier in this
paper, it is easy to conclude that spiritual experiences and religious beliefs are two related but
distinct terms. Spiritual experience is a very *personal* encounter that is out of the ordinary, often
a result of intense meditation or rhythmic rituals. Religious belief, on the other hand, is a faith or
creed of a divine deity (or deities) that relates to the *values* and *practices* based on teachings
within a *group* of people. The major problem with Neurotheology is that it confuses spiritual
experiences with religious beliefs.[2] "When these people talk of religious experience, they are
talking of a meditative experience," said John Haught, a professor of theology at Georgetown
University. "But religion is more than that. It involves commitments and suffering and struggle –
it's not all meditative bliss. It also involves moments when you feel abandoned by God. It is
symbolism and myth and story and much richer things. They have isolated one small aspect of
religious experience and they are identifying that with the whole of religion".[27]

Religious belief and faith are larger than the sum of our brain parts. Daniel Batson, a University
of Kansas psychologist who studies the effect of religion on people, describes the brain as "the
hardware through which religion is experienced". He further illustrates this with the analogy of
piano and music. To say that the brain produces religious beliefs is like saying "a piano produces
music".[27] Similarly, religious beliefs can be experienced via the brain, but encompasses more
than just spiritual experiences alone. Another very cool analogy is given by Professor Michael
McClymond. "A kiss," he says, "is more than a mutually agreed-upon exchange of saliva, breath

and germs".[27] All these illustrations serve to support the same point—that spiritual experience is only a small portion of religious beliefs, and does not equate to it. As such, even if experimental studies of the brain during meditation and prayer do show distinctively that spiritual experience is a mere creation of the brain (and I do not say that it has already been shown, as I have argued earlier), it still cannot be concluded that religious beliefs are created based on neurophysiological changes alone.

Yet, some would argue that although spiritual experience is not equivalent to religious beliefs, it is the root of religious beliefs. Humans are hard wired to *desire* and *need* spiritual experiences. It is because of this inherent yearning to feel such spiritual intensity that religions are created.

During meditation or prayer, the parietal lobe has decreased activity, leading to the sense of oneness with God and the universe. In addition to that, the temporal lobe is activated, which links experiences with personal significance. As a result, people who experience spiritually intense moments tend to relate the experience as a significant event in their lives, which thus leads to the belief in religion.[27]

Religion has existed across cultures for many generations, which is why people are interested in studying our need for religion, as well as why it can remain a need for so long. One possible explanation could lie in the causal operator of the brain. The causal operator makes us view reality in terms of causal sequences. It forces us to ask the "WHY" and "HOW" questions, such as why we exist, why something works the way it does, why an event happened, how the universe was created. Hence, the causal operator is highly responsible for scholarly pursuits in human science, philosophy and religion. Having a causal operator within our brain means that it is a biological necessity for us to seek out causality. Religious beliefs emerge as a result of our inherent need to find out the purpose of our existence, how the universe was created, as well as many other big questions that we have been unable to explain with our limited wisdom and knowledge. Religion is the only manner in which we can satisfy the causal operator which forces us to pose such difficult questions.[2, 28]

But, if religious beliefs are merely to answer to the causal operator that has been implanted in our brain, then how do non-religious people deal with the causal operator with nothing to appease it with?

One very prominent example of a person who has religious experiences but does not subscribe to any particular religious belief is Albert Einstein. Einstein was not conventionally religious. He rejected Judaism at the age of twelve, was doubtful of an afterlife, and did not believe in the existence of a God who cares, answers prayers, and judges when people die. Nonetheless, Einstein believed that "the most profound religious emotion that we can experience is the sensation of the mystical". Einstein believed in religious experiences, but had no religious beliefs to speak of.[17]

It cannot be said that religious experiences are the root of religious beliefs as they are not inseparable entities. There can be religious experiences without religious beliefs (as pointed out above), and there can also be religious beliefs without any religious experiences. Take the Aztecs for example. The Aztecs practice cannibalism, believing that victims that were sacrificed took on the nature of God. Thus, they believed that by eating the flesh of these victims, the power of God would be transferred to them. Similarly, the Binderwurs in India eat the dead to please the goddess Kali. Some African tribes ingest the bodies of enemies to ensure their ghosts have nowhere to live. Members of the Jivaro tribe remove, boil and dry the head of any killed enemy, believing that this ritual traps the spirit of the enemy within the head and prevents them seeking revenge. All these examples indicate that there does exist religious beliefs that do not have much linkage with spiritual experience, let alone be based upon it.[17, 29-30]

A common source of religious experience is rituals, but rituals definitely cannot be the source of religious beliefs. Ritualistic music and dance are widely practiced by many groups of people to induce religious experiences. The Ju/'hoansi in Botswana and Namibia sing and dance in circles after sunset, entering a trancelike state towards dawn; members of the Mevlevi sect of Islam chant the name of Allah as they perform an ecstatic dance; the Plains Indians practice the sun dance; voodoo believers invoke spirits by dancing.[17] However, rituals exist in non-human animals too. Bees dance; peacocks display; whales breech and flap their flukes.[28] Ritual behavior in non-human animals seems to be a way of overcoming social distance between individuals so that they can coordinate their activity in a way that would help the species survive. The rhythmic and repetitive nature of ritual stimulation, through ear, eye, or bodily motion, increases a sense of unity of purpose between individuals. Furthermore, it leads to coordinated arousal or discharge of the brain's limbic system, leading to a sense of profound unity within the participants.[12, 28] This is similar to what is observed in humans, where rituals that result in spiritual experiences cause the individual to lose sense of self and feel united with the community and the rest of the world. Thus, it seems that ritualizing is evolutionarily adaptive for many animals, and none more than the human. Some may say that this shows that rituals are but a need that is hard-wired in the human brain, just like it has been hard-wired into the brains of non-human animals. However, though non-human animals have rituals, they do not have religious beliefs. If rituals and the spiritual experiences that arise from rituals are the basis of religious beliefs, then why is it that humans practicing rituals have religious beliefs but non-human animals that practice rituals do not? To say that rituals (a common source of religious experience) are the basis of religious beliefs would imply that non-human animals should all have religious beliefs too, and this is utterly ridiculous. Henceforth, religious experiences cannot be said to be the root of religious beliefs and thus there cannot be any neurophysiological basis to religious beliefs.

The Brain evolved to create religious beliefs? Or Religious beliefs required the Brain to be that way?

Besides looking at science, people have also looked into history and evolution in the search of the origins of religious beliefs. It seems that the earliest records of religious beliefs and rituals occurred with the existence of the Upper Paleolithic people. Very coincidentally, it is also during this period of history that there seemed to be an emergence of a cognitively fluid mentality in humans.[31] Thus, by putting two and two together, the question is asked: Did the evolving of the human brain result in the emergence of religious beliefs?

Although such archeological evidences are concrete and cannot be invalidated, this argument for the evolving human brain as the basis of religious beliefs is only speculative. A discovery of religious records in the Upper Paleolithic People does not mean that humans before that period definitely had no religious beliefs. They could have had religious beliefs for all we know, just that there have been no records discovered, or they simply left no traces of it. This is not surprising, for more than 60,000 years have passed!

Thus far, all the so-called "evidences", be it scientific or archaeological, have only remained as speculative data in the claim that there is a neurophysiological basis for religious beliefs. From the opposite point of view, if a God (or gods) really exists, he would need a way for us to experience him, thus it is not unreasonable to have sections of the brain catered for spiritual experience. Being ultimately still human, we need to connect any deity or spiritual entity to a reference, based on our own experience and culture. We need to *humanize* God in our brain. It is a matter of outer world sensory stimuli versus an inner world of imaginative symbolizing. What we can imagine God as, is only but a symbolic form of who God really is, and to symbolize God into a personal language that we can understand does not make God into an object about which to argue. God is always more than our idea of God, simply because we have only the idea of the symbolic version of God that our brain has interpreted, but not the true complete God that exists.[32] An analogy by renegade biologist Rupert Sheldrake is very apt:

"If I switch on my TV set to PBS and if you measure different bits of the tuning set, you'll find that certain bits are resonating at certain frequencies. If I switch it to another channel, like Fox News, there will be measurable frequency changes in the various bits of the TV. But that doesn't prove that all the content of PBS programs and Fox News is generated inside that bit of the TV set. I think that the thinking behind a lot of neuroscience claims is as naïve as that, because it's based on the assumption that it's all inside the brain. Therefore the next question is: Which bits of the brain explain it? But if the brain is not like that, if the brain is more like a tuning system and a center for coordinating our actions and our sensations, then there's no reason to assume that all our mental activity is confined to the inside of the head." [40]

The brain is like a receiver or transmitter, a tool to help us understand our surroundings. It is a "cognitive prosthesis" for the soul, as developmental psychologist Paul Bloom puts it.[40]

With so many people scrambling to investigate the brain and the way it works, we sometimes get so caught up with the minute details that we forget the big picture. All these neurophysiology that has been detected and analyzed in the human brain definitely serve a big part in understanding how the brain works. What is missing, though, is that there is more to it—the cause or origin of these neuron firings. Using Templeton prize–winning cosmologist George Ellis's illustration, we seem to be too engrossed in looking at the brain from a bottom-up view, and missing the top-down approach totally. Think of a jumbo jet. The bottom-up view of why it flies is understood by the action of particles impacting the wings from below as opposed to those from above, thus giving it an uplift and thrust that keeps the plane flying in the air. The top-down approach, on the other hand, understands that the plane flies because someone designed it to be that way. The mistake with fundamentalists is that they tend to focus deeply on the partial cause rather than the whole cause. Unquestionably, the brain is there and the neurons are firing. But that is only a partial cause of our experiences, and there is more to religious beliefs than just mere firings of the brain.[40]

Conclusion

The human study of the neurophysiological reactions in religious experiences does not reductively negate the existence of God. Rather, it only serves to investigate the mechanisms involved in the process of us humanizing God using our brain, for our own understanding. It is a study of how the divine is translated into the human realm; a conceptualization from the archetypal to the material world. This human capacity to experience the divine is natural, just as we have a capacity to comprehend language and mathematics. I quote Antonio Damasio, "To discover that a particular feeling [including any feeling involved in responding to God] depends on activity in a number of specific brain systems interacting with a number of body organs does not diminish the status of that feeling as a human phenomenon. Neither anguish nor the elation that love or art can bring about [is] devalued by understanding some of the myriad biological processes that make them what they are. Precisely the opposite should be true: Our sense of wonder should increase before the intricate mechanisms that make such magic possible".[12] Neuroscience has undoubtedly progressed very far, but it still cannot answer the epistemological question of whether God made the brain or the brain made God. The brain may be wired to receive religious feelings, but the claim that there is a neurophysiological *basis* for religious beliefs has no support and thus does not stand.

References

1. Sharon Begley. (2001). *Searching For the God Within. The way our brains are wired may explain the origin and power of religious beliefs*. Newsweek Magazine/January 29
2. Newberg, A. B., E. G. d'Aquili, and V. P. Rause. (2001). *Why God Won't Go Away: Brain Science and the Biology of Belief*. New York: Ballantine.
3. http://en.wikipedia.org/wiki/Religious_belief
4. Habel, Norman, O'Donoghue, Michael and Maddox, Marion. (1993). 'Religious experience'. In: *Myth, ritual and the sacred. Introducing the phenomena of religion* Underdale: University of South Australia
5. Charlesworth, Max. (1988). *Religious experience. Unit A. Study guide 2*. Deakin University
6. http://en.wikipedia.org/wiki/Religious_experience
7. Andrew Newberg. (2001). *Pathological and Normal Spiritual Experiences* http://www.metanexus.net/magazine/tabid/68/id/8523/Default.aspx
8. Andrew Nerberg. (2001). *Defining the Self.* http://www.metanexus.net/magazine/tabid/68/id/8521/Default.aspx
9. Iona Miller. (2003). *How the Brain 'Creates' God. The Emerging Science of Neurotheology*. Asklepia Foundation.
10. Damasio, Antonio. (1994). *Descartes' Error: Emotion, Reason and the Human Brain*. New York: G. P. Putnam's Sons.
11. Kandel, Eric R., James H. Schwartz, and Thomas M. Jessell, eds. (2000). *Principles of Neural Scien*ce (4th. ed.). New York: McGraw-Hill
12. Cliff Guthrie. *Neurology, Ritual, and Religion: An Initial Exploration. Or: "Were you there when they stimulated our amygdalas? Sometimes it causes me to tremble"*. 2000
13. Andrew Newberg. (2001). *Reality from the Inside* http://www.metanexus.net/magazine/tabid/68/id/8522/Default.aspx
14. Sharon Begley. (2001). *Your Brain on Religion: Mystic visions or brain circuits at work?* In the new field of "neurotheology," scientists seek the biological basis of spirituality. Is God all in our heads? Newsweek Magazine/May 7
15. Mandell, A. J. (1980). *Toward a psychobiology of transcendence: God in the brain*. In J. M. Davidson, & R. J. Davidson (Eds.), The Psychobiology of Consciousness. New York: Plenum.
16. Wright, P. A. (1989). *The nature of the shamanic state of consciousness: A review*. Journal of Psychoactive Drugs, 21 (1), 25-33.
17. Dean Hamer. (2004). *The God Gene: How Faith is Hardwired into our genes*. A Division of Random House, Inc., New York. Chapters 2, 4, 7.

18. Doblin, R. (1991). *Pahnke's Good Friday Experiment: A Long Term Follow-up and Methodological Critique.* J Transpers Psychology. 23
19. Shankar Vedantam. (2001). *Tracing the Synapses of Our Spirituality: Researchers Examine Relationship Between Brain and Religion.*
20. Bear, D. M. (1979). *Temporal lobe epilepsy—a syndrome of sensory-limbic hyperconnection.* Cortex 15: 357-384.
21. Bear, D. M., & Fedio, P. (1977). *Quantitative analysis of interictal behavior in temporal lobe epilepsy.* Archives of Neurology, 34, 454–467.
22. Saver, J. L., & Rabin, J. (1997). *The neural substrates of religious experience.* Journal of Neuropsychiatry and Clinical Neurosciences, 9, 498–510.
23. Ramachandran V.S. (1998). *Phantoms in the Brain: Human Nature and the Architecture of the Mind.* Fourth Estate
24. Eliade. (1964). *Shamanism: Archaic Technics of Fantasy.* New York: Pantheon.
25. Tucker, D. M., Novelly, R. A.,&Walker, P. J. (1987). *Hyperreligiosity in temporal lobe epilepsy: Redefining the relationship.* Journal of Nervous and Mental Disorders, 175, 181–184.
26. Henrik Ehrsson et al. (2005). *Neural substrate of body size: illusory feeling of shrinking of the waist.* PLoS. 3(12): e412.
27. Shankar Vedantam. (2001). *Tracing the Synapses of Our Spirituality: Researchers Examine Relationship Between Brain and Religion.*
28. d'Aquili and Newberg. (1999). *The Mystical Mind: Probing the Biology of Religious Experience.* Fortress Press, Minneapolis.
29. Morris B. (1987). *Anthropological Studies of Religion: An Introductory Text.* Cambridge, UK: The Cambridge University Press.
30. Gibson, A., D. Simpson. (1998). *Prehistoric Ritual and Religion.* Gloucestershire, UK: Sutton Publishing Ltd.
31. Steven Mithen. (1996). *Prehistory of the Mind.* Thames and Hudson Ltd., London. Chapter 9.
32. Albright C.R. and Ashbrook J.B. (2001). *Where God lives in the human brain.* Sourcebooks, Inc. Naperville, Illinois. Chapters 2, 7.
33. Newberg, A. and Lee, B. (2005). *The neuroscientific study of religious and spiritual phenomena: or why God doesn't use biostatistics.* Zygon. 40(2), 469-489.
34. Lou, H. C., T. W. Kjaer, L. Friberg, G. Wildschiodtz, S. Holm, and M. Nowak. (1999). *A 15O-H2O PET Study of Meditation and the Resting State of Normal Consciousness.* Human Brain Mapping 7 (2): 98–105.
35. Newberg, A., Alavi, A., Baime, M. et al. (2001). *Measurement of regional cerebral blood flow during the complex cognitive task of meditation: a preliminary SPECT study.* Psychiatr Res Neuroimaging. 106, 113-122.
36. Newberg, A. and Iversen, J. (2003). *The neural basis of the complex mental task of meditation: neurotransmitter and neurochemical considerations.* Medical Hypotheses. 51(2), 282-291.
37. D'Aquili, E.G. and Newberg, A. (2000). *The Neuropsychology of Aesthetic, Spiritual and Mystical States.* Zygon. 35(1), 39-51.
38. Ring, K. (1980). *Life at Death: A Scientific Investigation of the Near-Death Experience.* New York: Quill.

39. Sim, M. K., and W. F. Tsoi. (1992). *The Effects of Centrally Acting Drugs on the EEG Correlates of Meditation.* Biofeedback and Self-Regulation. 17, 215–20.
40. Hamilton, C. (2005). *Is God all in Your Head? Inside science's quest to solve the mystery of consciousness.* What is Enlightenment? Issue 29.